CONTENTS

GW00728153

INTRODUCTION

The greatest love that a human being can ever experience is the unconditional love of God our Father in heaven. The very definition of God is that He is Love.

God's love is not self-seeking. God the Father does not love us because of what He can get from us. Instead, He shows us His love by bestowing His heavenly blessings upon us and upon our lives.

He that loveth not knoweth not God; for God is love.

1 JOHN 4:8

I am writing this book to introduce you to the deep and immeasurable love of God that is waiting for you. His arms are outstretched and ready to embrace you. He wants to bring you closer to Himself so that you can experience the fullness of this divine love. It will transform your life forever, as it did mine.

As you read this book, open up your heart and receive His love for you. I see you receiving unconditional love in Jesus name!

CHAPTER 1

NO ONE IS TOO BAD, TOO EVIL OR TOO WICKED TO RECEIVE THE FATHER'S LOVE

When we think about all the bad things we have done in our lives, we can easily condemn ourselves. Some feel so worthless that they commit suicide because they have lost all hope and they think that there is no place of forgiveness for them.

If you are feeling hopeless, I am announcing to you right now that the Father's heart is bursting with love and forgiveness for you. It does not matter what you have done. He does not care how many abortions you have committed. He does not care if you are the head of a gang. He does not care if you are a drug addict. He does not care if you have murdered before.

I will say it again, it does not matter what you have done. No sin is so appalling that the love of God our Father cannot reach and forgive. The word of God says that while we were sinners, God sent His son to come and die for us and pay the penalty for all our sins.

But God commendeth his love toward us, in that, while we were yet sinners, Christ died for us.

ROMANS 5:8

This is truly love that we do not deserve. You see, as human beings we tend to love for selfish reasons. We often love others because of what we can get from them. It may be because of your money, your looks or even your passport that someone loves you.

But as soon as that thing is not available, they will turn away from you. Our heavenly Father is not like that. The cardinal sign of God's love towards us is that He gives only His best to us.

CHAPTER 2

SALVATION:
THE FATHER'S GREATEST
LOVE TO HUMANITY

In the beginning, God created the heavens and the earth. He gave to mankind the dominion, power and authority to govern the earth. But mankind lost this relationship with the Father through sin. Because of sin, we lost our position, our power and our authority to govern the earth to the devil.

And God said, Let us make man in our image, after our likeness: and let them have dominion over the fish of the sea, and over the fowl of the air, and over the cattle, and over all the earth, and over every creeping thing that creepeth upon the earth.

GENESIS 1:26

When man sinned, man died spiritually. This meant that his relationship with God was cut short. This is the reason why we need salvation. Salvation restores our relationship with God our Father.

Since the fall of man, God has been seeking to restore His relationship with mankind. To prove it, God gave us the greatest gift of all. He sent His only son to die for our sins. For this reason, whosoever receives His son Jesus Christ shall no longer live in sin and perish but shall have eternal life.

For God so loved the world, that he gave his only begotten Son, that whosoever believeth in him should not perish, but have everlasting life. For God sent not his Son into the world to condemn the world; but that the world through him might be saved.

JOHN 3:16-17

God our Father paid the ultimate price to redeem mankind to Himself. We were all destined to die and condemned to death by sin. The only payment for our sin was a life for a life and God our Father paid it through His son Jesus Christ. The death of Jesus Christ on the cross is mankind's freedom into eternal life.

God is calling you today to receive this free gift that He gave to all of humanity so that you will not go to hell when you die. God wants to exchange the life of His son Jesus Christ for your life so that you can experience the fullness of His love here on earth.

He wants to take all your mistakes, disappointments, sins, shortcomings and poverty and in return give you all His goodness and His blessings.

His word is true. No matter how deep your sins are, if you call on the name of the Lord you shall be saved.

And it shall come to pass, that whosoever shall call on the name of the Lord shall be saved.

ACTS 2:21

CHAPTER 3

HOW CAN I RECEIVE THE
LOVE OF THE FATHER?

The word of God tells us that whosoever shall call on the name of the Lord shall be saved. Whosoever means whosoever.

For there is no difference between the Jew and the Greek: for the same Lord over all is rich unto all that call upon him. For whosoever shall call upon the name of the Lord shall be saved.

ROMANS 10:12-13

You and I are the 'whosoever' that Jesus Christ came to die for. It does not matter how deep your sins are, the blood of Jesus can wash it away! There is no sin that God cannot forgive, there is no sin under heaven that the blood of Jesus cannot wash.

For God so loved the world, that he gave his only begotten Son, that whosoever believeth in him should not perish, but have everlasting life.

JOHN 3:16

God has already paid the price for you by sacrificing a life for you. This life is the life of Jesus that has been sacrificed for you for eternity. In fact, Jesus bought you from satan with His life. Once you accept Jesus Christ, satan no longer has the right to interfere with your life and take you to hell.

If you want to accept Jesus Christ as your Lord and Saviour, you as the individual must acknowledge that you are a sinner and repent of your sins. True repentance is of the heart. Jesus said that unless a man is born again he cannot see the kingdom of God.

There is only one way to be born again and receive salvation and that is through Jesus Christ. All others are liars. Jesus said, *I am the way, the truth and the life: no man cometh unto the Father but by Me (John 14:6).* Jesus also said, *I am the door (John 10:9).* Even the very door to heaven is Jesus!

My friend, do not be deceived by the doctrine of devils being preached by some prominent people you may know because one day they will all bow before the King of kings and the Lord of lords.

I have often heard people say "I am a good person and so I will go to heaven". But be not deceived, you can never be good enough for heaven. It is not by our own works but by the mercy and love of God.

The truth is that you cannot be saved by your own works *(Ephesians 2:8,9).* In fact, all our good deeds are like filthy rags before the Lord. You can be very loving, you can be extremely kind, you can give all your money to the poor, you can establish many charities to help mankind. You can pay tithes, sing in the choir and even preach but all these cannot save you. There is no such thing as being too good to go to hell!

For we ourselves also were sometimes foolish, disobedient, deceived, serving divers lusts and pleasures, living in malice and envy, hateful, and hating one another.
But after that the kindness and love of God our Saviour toward man appeared, Not by works of righteousness which we have done, but according to his mercy he saved us, by the washing of regeneration, and renewing of the Holy Ghost; Which he shed on us abundantly through Jesus Christ our Saviour.

TITUS 3:3-6

The word of God also tells us in Acts 4:12 that apart from Jesus, there is no other name under heaven by which we must be saved. In other words, there is no salvation in any other name except the name of Jesus Christ.

Now, if you will confess Jesus Christ with your mouth and believe in your heart that God has raised Him from the dead, you shall be saved. It is as simple as that!

You just have to believe it with all your heart and confess with your mouth that Jesus is Lord *(Romans 10:9,10)*.

When you become born again or saved, God our Father gives you a new heart. Your heart is created again and you become a new person. All your sins are washed away by the precious blood of Jesus. Jesus makes everything new. It is as though your past never existed. You become a new creature and you can no longer be condemned by your past.

Therefore if any man be in Christ, he is a new creature: old things are passed away; behold, all things are become new.

2 CORINTHIANS 5:17

As soon as you receive Jesus into your life you are transported from the kingdom of darkness, which is the devil's kingdom, into the kingdom of light, which is God's kingdom *(Colossians 1:13)*. The Lord now gives you power to become His royal son or daughter. You are now adopted into the family of God. Hallelujah!

CHAPTER 4

SALVATION vs BAPTISM

People sometimes confuse being born again or saved, with water baptism. They think that being baptised is the same as being born again.

But I tell you the truth, if a person is not born again and they get baptised, the baptism does not make the person saved. That person has only been washed with water and nothing spiritual has taken place in his or her heart. Salvation is of the heart and water baptism alone does not reach the heart. After all we bath everyday!

I was both baptised and confirmed whilst I was in secondary school. The reason why I decided to do both baptism and confirmation was so that I never had to do them again.

But I was wrong. I was wrong because I was not saved before the baptism and confirmation. So after the baptism and confirmation, there was no change in my life. I did not know the Lord; neither did I have a relationship with Him. I was an unsaved soul washed with drinking water.

However, two years after this event, I received the Lord Jesus Christ as my Saviour into my heart and became truly born again. I was then baptised again, but this time, I felt the presence of the Holy Spirit upon my life while I was coming out of the water. I became a born again, Holy Spirit filled, tongue speaking believer.

Jesus said, *except a man be born of water and of the Spirit he cannot enter into the kingdom of God (John 3:5)*. The word 'water' in this verse has nothing to do with baptism but it is talking about the word of God which is able to save our souls. According to 1 Peter 1:23, we become born again by the word of God. Read it for yourself.

Being born again, not of corruptible seed, but of incorruptible, by the word of God, which liveth and abideth for ever.

1 PETER 1:23

We therefore do not become born again by water baptism. We are not saved by water baptism. Ephesians 5:26 makes this even clearer as it refers to the word of God as water.

That he might sanctify and cleanse it with the washing of water by the word.

EPHESIANS 5:26

You can now see that if you are baptised with water and you are not saved by the word of God, then you are deceiving yourself by thinking that you are saved.

Baptism comes from the Greek word Baptiso which means 'whelm' or 'to fully submerge'. It does not mean sprinkling of water. The baptism that I did in secondary school was sprinkling of water and it made no difference in my life.

Let's get it right. Jesus Christ is our best example and we must imitate Him in all aspects of our Christian life. We must allow the word of God to guide us and not follow the traditions of men. Jesus himself was baptised by John the Baptist in the river Jordan and He was fully immersed in the water.

Then cometh Jesus from Galilee to Jordan unto John, to be baptized of him. But John forbad him, saying, I have need to be baptized of thee, and comest thou to me?
And Jesus answering said unto him, Suffer it to be so now: for thus it becometh us to fulfil all righteousness. Then he suffered him. And Jesus, when he was baptized, went up straightway out of the water: and, lo, the heavens were opened unto him, and he saw the Spirit of God descending like a dove, and lighting upon him:
And lo a voice from heaven, saying, This is my beloved Son, in whom I am well pleased.

MATTHEW 3:13-17

In the above passage of scripture, you can see that Jesus came out of the river Jordan. Therefore he was fully immersed in the water. He even came out of the water praying *(Luke 3:21)*.

Now in the mouth of two or three shall every word be established so I will give a second example. Apart from the example of Jesus' baptism, the disciple named Philip also baptised the Ethiopian eunuch.

In an amazing passage of scripture in Acts 8:26-40, the Ethiopian eunuch requested that Philip baptise him. But look at what Philip said to him. Philip said, *"If thou believest with all thine heart"*. The Ethiopian eunuch was born again before being baptised fully in water. Read it for yourself.

And the angel of the Lord spake unto Philip, saying, Arise, and go toward the south unto the way that goeth down from Jerusalem unto Gaza, which is desert.

And he arose and went: and, behold, a man of Ethiopia, an eunuch of great authority under Candace queen of the Ethiopians, who had the charge of all her treasure, and had come to Jerusalem for to worship, Was returning, and sitting in his chariot read Esaias the prophet.

Then the Spirit said unto Philip, Go near, and join thyself to this chariot. And Philip ran thither to him, and heard him read the prophet Esaias, and said, Understandest thou what thou readest? And he said, How can I, except some man should guide me? And he desired Philip that he would come up and sit with him.

The place of the scripture which he read was this, He was led as a sheep to the slaughter; and like a lamb dumb before his shearer, so opened he not his mouth: In his humiliation his judgment was taken away: and who shall declare his generation? for his life is taken from the earth.

And the eunuch answered Philip, and said, I pray thee, of whom speaketh the prophet this? of himself, or of some other man?

Then Philip opened his mouth, and began at the same scripture, and preached unto him Jesus.

And as they went on their way, they came unto a certain water: and the eunuch said, See, here is water; what doth hinder me to be baptized? And Philip said, If thou believest with all thine heart, thou mayest. And he answered and said, I believe that Jesus Christ is the Son of God.

And he commanded the chariot to stand still: and they went down both into the water, both Philip and the eunuch; and he baptized him. And when they were come up out of the water, the Spirit of the Lord caught away Philip, that the eunuch saw him no more: and he went on his way rejoicing. But Philip was found at Azotus: and passing through he preached in all the cities, till he came to Caesarea.

ACTS 8:26-40

Nevertheless, water baptism is still very significant. Water baptism is symbolic of our death and resurrection with Jesus Christ. It is also our public declaration that we are saved.

The lowering of the person in water signifies our death with Jesus Christ and the raising of the person out of the water symbolises our resurrection with Jesus Christ.

Therefore we are buried with him by baptism into death: that like as Christ was raised up from the dead by the glory of the Father, even so we also should walk in newness of life. For if we have been planted together in the likeness of his death, we shall be also in the likeness of his resurrection.

ROMANS 6:4-5

Once you are born again you can get baptised in the sea or in a swimming pool. The most important thing is to do the baptism as Jesus did. He was baptised by being fully immersed in the water.

PRAYER OF SALVATION

If you are reading this book and you want to experience this divine love of God our Father, it starts with just one step. Surrender your life to Jesus today and restore your eternal relationship with God our Father.

Please say this simple prayer:

My Father in heaven, I recognise that I am a sinner. I recognise that the Lord Jesus died for me and paid the penalty of my sins.

Dear Lord, today I repent of my sins and I accept Jesus Christ as my Lord and my Saviour. Wash me with your blood and make me holy.

Please write my name in the book of life and give me the grace to serve you for the rest of my life.

Thank you that I am born again.

Amen.

CHAPTER 5

WHAT MUST I DO
NOW THAT I AM SAVED?

Congratulations! You are now a new creation in Christ! The very first step to take is to get yourself a good Christian Bible and start reading it so that your heavenly Father can begin to teach you His wonderful word.

As you read His word, you will get to know Him and fellowship with Him. Start reading the Bible from the book of John chapter 1. It will give you a solid understanding of what the word of God is and the love that the Father has for you.

Secondly, find a good Bible believing church where the

pure word of God is taught and attend regularly. This will help you to grow and be firmly established in God's kingdom.

Thirdly, develop a regular habit of daily prayer. Having a prayerful life means that you fellowship with the Lord every morning like David did in the book of Psalms and it builds your relationship with the Lord.

My voice shalt thou hear in the morning, O LORD; in the morning will I direct my prayer unto thee, and will look up.

PSALMS 5:3

During this time of prayer and fellowship, read your Bible after praying. Have a little notebook with you and write down whatever the Lord tells you.

Lastly, be aware that there is the danger of going back to your past life. Invite your friends to also receive Jesus Christ and ask God for the grace to never go back to your past life. If you keep hanging out with the same friends you used to do bad things with, it will be difficult to stay focused on God.

Wherefore come out from among them, and be ye separate, saith the Lord, and touch not the unclean thing; and I will receive you, And will be a Father unto you, and ye shall be my sons and daughters, saith the Lord Almighty.

2 CORINTHIANS 6:17-18

If those friends refuse to come with you, you will have to make a decision to cut them out of your new life in Christ and make new friends in the kingdom of God.

I am so happy that you are saved!

The angels of heaven are all rejoicing at this very moment and singing in the presence of the Living God. They are rejoicing because of your salvation!

I welcome you into this marvellous family of God. Walk with the Lord and truly serve Him all the days of your life.

God bless you.

ABOUT THE AUTHOR

Reverend Ernest Addo is the Founder and Senior Pastor of Living Jesus Tabernacle, based in London, UK. His transforming ministry is characterised by the manifest works of the Holy Spirit and his forthright preaching and teaching of the word of God.

As a seasoned church planter, missionary and author, Rev. Ernest has a burning passion for lost souls to be saved. He was trained by Bishop Dag Heward-Mills and ordained into the ministry by Pastor Benny Hinn. He is also a member of World Healing Fellowship of which Pastor Benny Hinn is the president.

Rev. Ernest holds a master's degree in information systems management and a bachelor's degree in publishing studies. He is happily married to his lovely wife Pastor Angella, who stands with him in his global vision for the ministry.

BOOKS BY REV. ERNEST ADDO
Three Dimensions of Man
The Foundations of True Faith
Meeting and Knowing the Holy Spirit
Spiritual Emergency
How to Pray: 60 Minutes in His Presence
The Father's Love

If you wish to order copies, please contact
ERNEST ADDO MINISTRIES
TEL: +44 07583 567 944
EMAIL: ernestaddoministries@gmail.com

LIVING JESUS TABERNACLE

Living Jesus Tabernacle (LJT) is a church
that is on fire for Jesus.

We would be delighted to support and encourage you
in your new life in Jesus Christ. Join us for one of our
services or check us out online – see details below.

We look forward to welcoming you!

You can VISIT us:
Sundays at 10am & Wednesdays at 7:30pm
Living Jesus Tabernacle
Forest Gate Community School
Forest Lane, Forest Gate
London, E7 9BB
UK

You can follow us on FACEBOOK:
www.facebook.com/LivingJesusTabernacle
You can CALL us:
+44 07583 567 944
You can EMAIL us:
livingjesustabernacle@gmail.com

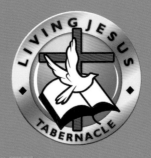

THE
FATHER'S
LOVE

Rev. Ernest Addo

The greatest love that a human being can ever experience
is the unconditional love of God our Father in heaven.
The very definition of God is that He is Love. As you
read this book, open your heart and receive The Father's
Love that is waiting just for you.

9 780993 225024

CTS Explanations
CTS Explanations
CTS Explanations

Explaining Catholic Teaching

Euthanasia

by Philip Robinson

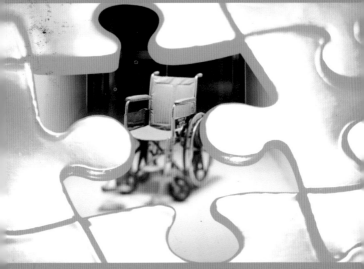

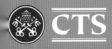

CTS Publications

CTS booklets explain the faith, teaching and life of the Catholic Church. They are based on Sacred Scripture, the Second Vatican Council documents, and the *Catechism of the Catholic Church*. Our booklets provide authentic Catholic teaching; they address issues of life and of truth which are relevant to all. They aim to inform and educate readers on the many issues that people have to deal with today.

In addition, CTS nurtures and supports the Christian life through its many spiritual, liturgical, educational and pastoral books. As Publisher to the Holy See, CTS publishes the official documents of the Catholic Church as they are issued.

website: www.cts-online.org.uk

ISBN 1 86082 191 X

Front cover image: compiled from two sources. *Jigsaw image*, Tom Lang copyright © Tom Lang/CORBIS Stock Market. *Wheelchair image* copyright © Corbis images.